THE COMPLETE VITAMINS AND MINERALS POCKET GUIDE

GEORGE MIHALACHE

DEDICATION

This book is dedicated to my F.I.R.E. (Financial Independence and Early Retirement) movement - U.K. friends, known and unknown.

George C. Mihalache

CONTENTS

ACKNOWLEDGMENTS

Special thanks to Huw Davies, who give me the idea for this book, and to my brother, for his input in writing it faster. Thank you to all who helped me with the research part, too.

Chapter 1

VITAMINS

George C. Mihalache

1. VITAMINS

INTRODUCTION

Vitamins do not share a common chemistry, but they do share certain characteristics. They are all organic nutrients that are necessary in small amounts for normal body functioning and good health. A well-balanced diet should provide most of the vitamins people need to stay healthy and prevent disease. Vitamin D is the only exception. Supplements can be helpful in some situations, such as pregnancy and certain illnesses. Strict vegetarians may benefit from taking vitamin B12 supplements. Unlike carbohydrates, fats, and proteins, vitamins are not sources of energy. Instead, vitamins are involved in the body's metabolism, cell production, tissue repair, and other vital processes. If you want to know more about, read this book. Find if you are one of the people who need them and why.

Vitamins are either fat soluble or water soluble. Fat-soluble vitamins, which include A, D, E, and K, are stored in the liver and used up by the body very slowly. Because the body stores fat-soluble vitamins, they can be dangerous when taken in large amounts. Water-soluble vitamins include vitamin C and the B vitamins. The body uses these vitamins very quickly. Excess amounts are removed in the urine. The Recommended Dietary Allowance (RDA) for vitamins, set by the Food and Nutrition Board of the National Academy of Sciences-National Research Council, has been used for years as a guide for determining the amount of vitamins needed to prevent deficiency diseases. The RDA is an estimate of the average requirements of dietary components such as calories, vitamins, minerals, and proteins that are needed to prevent deficiency. Different groups of people need different amounts of vitamins based on their gender and age.

The RDA is gradually being replaced by a new standard

called the Dietary Reference Intake (DRI). The DRI is a general term used to describe the types and amounts of nutrients healthy people need.

The DRI values are based on four categories:

- The **recommended dietary allowance (RDA)**. This is the current rating on most vitamins. An RDA is the average daily dietary intake level; sufficient to meet the nutrient requirements of nearly all (97-98 percent) healthy individuals in a group. It is calculated from an **Estimated Average Requirement (EAR).** If sufficient scientific evidence is not available to establish an EAR, and thus calculate an RDA, an AI is usually developed. -The estimated average requirement (EAR). This is the amount of the vitamin needed to meet the nutritional requirements for 50% of the population. An Estimated Average Requirement (EAR) is the average daily nutrient intake level estimated to meet the requirements of half of the healthy individuals in a group. EARs have not been established for vitamin K, pantothenic acid, biotin, choline, chromium, fluoride, manganese, or other nutrients not yet evaluated via the DRI process.

- **Adequate intake (AI)**. This amount is used if there are not enough data to calculate the RDA. For healthy breastfed infants, an AI is the mean intake. The AI for other life stage and gender groups is believed to cover the needs of all healthy individuals in the groups, but lack of data or uncertainty in the data prevent being able to specify with confidence the percentage of individuals covered by this intake. See RDA definition

- **Tolerable upper intake level (UL).** This is the maximum dose that is likely to be safe in 98% of the population. A Tolerable Upper Intake Level (UL) is the highest level of daily nutrient intake that is likely to pose no risk of adverse health effects to almost all individuals in the general population. Unless otherwise specified, the UL represents total intake from food, water, and supplements. Due to a lack of suitable data, ULs could not be established for vitamin K, thiamin, riboflavin, vitamin B12, pantothenic acid, biotin, and carotenoids. In the absence of a UL, extra caution may be warranted in consuming levels above recommended intakes.

Members of the general population should be advised not to routinely exceed the UL. The UL is not meant to apply to individuals who are treated with the nutrient under medical supervision or to individuals with predisposing conditions that modify their sensitivity to the nutrient.

Dietary supplement use is on the rise. More than half of American adults use supplements, most often multivitamins and minerals. In particular, more Americans are taking vitamin D and calcium supplements than in the past. However, studies have found no difference in mortality rates between people who take vitamin supplements and those who don't take supplements. Most people who eat a healthy diet do not need vitamins, but there are some exceptions.

1. **Pregnant and Breastfeeding Women**. Women who are pregnant or breastfeeding will generally need additional vitamins. Folic acid, vitamins B6 and B12 are particularly important during pregnancy. Women who are vegetarians need to take enough of vitamin B12. A deficiency in this vitamin can harm their baby. Folic acid reduces the risk for neural tube defects and possibly deformities of the face, such as cleft palate. Studies also link low folate levels during pregnancy with low birth weight, which may increase the risk of heart disease in adulthood. A woman's best approach is to start taking extra folic acid plus multivitamin supplements before she becomes pregnant. The human body stores several years' worth of vitamin B12, so deficiency of this vitamin is extremely rare. However, people who follow a strict vegetarian diet and do not eat eggs or dairy products may need to take vitamin B12 supplements. Pregnant women who eat a healthy diet may still have low folate levels and need to take folic acid supplements. Requirements are as follows: The recommended dietary allowance (RDA) for folic acid before getting pregnant is 400 mcg. During pregnancy the RDA is 600 mcg. Women who are breast-feeding should get 500 mcg of folic acid. Some women have low vitamin A reserves in their liver. However, getting too much vitamin A from food or supplements significantly increases the risk for birth defects. Experts recommend that

pregnant women get no more than 3,000 mcg of vitamin A each day.

2. **Infants and Children**. Infants who are breastfed by healthy mothers should receive enough vitamins. However, in some cases, infants may not get enough of vitamins K and D. Human milk contains low levels of vitamin K, and the newborn's immature intestinal tract may not produce enough of the baby's own supply. Most babies are given an injection of this vitamin at birth. Infants who are breast-fed by malnourished women or who do not get enough sunlight exposure may be deficient in vitamin D. In these cases, supplements of 200 - 300 IU are recommended. Formulas are required to contain enough vitamins and minerals. After infancy, most American children receive all the vitamins they need from their diet, unless they are severely deprived. However, research suggests that many healthy children ages 1 to 11, especially African-American and Hispanic children, are not getting enough vitamin D.

3. **Smokers**. Smoking interferes with the absorption of several vitamins, especially vitamins C and D. Smoking can also interfere with the metabolism of vitamin D, resulting in poor muscle function. Taking supplements of antioxidant vitamins, especially beta-carotene, is harmful to smokers. Instead of taking supplements, smokers should eat a diet rich in fresh fruits, vegetables, and whole grains. Smoking cessation is the most important intervention.

4. **Alcoholics**. Alcoholics often have several vitamin deficiencies. The most dangerous deficiencies are: Vitamin B1 (thiamin), Vitamin B2 (riboflavin), Vitamin B6 (pyridoxine), Folic acid, Vitamin C. Low levels of vitamin B6 may increase the risk for colorectal cancer in men who drink large amounts of alcohol.

5. **People who have had gastric bypass surgery**. Vitamin deficiency is a complication of gastric bypass surgery. Women, African-Americans, and adults who have

had laparoscopic Roux-en-Y bypass surgery are at highest risk. The deficiency is treated with water-soluble vitamin supplements.

6. **Strict Vegetarians**. Strict vegetarians need to take vitamin B12 supplements, unless they get enough of this vitamin from fortified cereals and other grain products. They may also need to take vitamin D and riboflavin supplements, or a multivitamin, and watch their iron levels. Vegans, who do not eat dairy, eggs, fish or meat may be at risk for vitamin A deficiencies if they do not eat plenty of dark-colored fruits and vegetables. Vitamin deficiencies may be particularly harmful in vegetarian children. Pregnant and breastfeeding women who are vegetarians must get enough vitamins. Mothers who do not get enough vitamin B12 may cause growth and nervous system problems in their newborns.

7. **People who are often on a diet**. People who are on weight-reduction diets of fewer than 1,000 calories a day should probably take a multivitamin. They should also check in regularly with a physician to make sure they are getting enough nutrients.

8. **Older Adults**. Almost a third of elderly people do not get enough of certain vitamins and important minerals. Often their dietary habits slip and they fail to regularly eat balanced meals. In addition, older adults are more likely to take medications that prevent the absorption of certain vitamins.

Common vitamin deficiencies in the elderly: Elderly people, particularly if they are not exposed to sunlight, may be deficient in vitamin D. Older adults should get at least 800 IU of vitamin D a day. People who are obese, or who have osteoporosis, limited sun exposure, or poor nutrient absorption may need to increase their intake to as much as 2,000 IU per day. Seniors also may have low levels of important B vitamins. Older adults with symptoms of dementia should be tested for a B12 deficiency. Seniors need to use caution when taking vitamin supplements. Because metabolism slows with age, it takes the liver longer to remove vitamins from the body. Therefore, the effect of some vitamin supplements may be intensified in older adults. For example, a dose of vitamin A that might be harmless in a younger adult could be toxic in an elderly patient.

9. **People Who Avoid Sunlight.** People who avoid sunlight or who are housebound, and whose diet is low in foods that contain vitamin D should take supplements. People with darker skin are at higher risk for vitamin D deficiencies than those with whiter skin. (Note: Vitamin D is toxic in high doses, and no one should exceed the RDI of vitamin D except under a physician's direction.)

Vitamin A

Known as retinol, axerophthol, biosterol, anti-infective vitamin. Present in supplements and used in food fortifications as retinyl palmitate and retinyl acetate. First isolated in 1913 by two groups of American workers. One microgram retinol = 3.3 international units (i.u.). Found only in foods of animal origin, but its active precursor beta-carotene is present in fruits and vegetables.

Vitamin A (micrograms/d)				
Age		EAR	RDA/AI	UL
	0-6mo	N/A	400*	600
Infant	6-12mo	N/A	500*	600
	1-3y	210	300	600
Children	4-8y	275	400	900
	9-13y	445	600	1700
	14-18y	630	900	2800
	19-30y	625	900	3000
	31-50y	625	900	3000
	51-70y	625	900	3000
Males	>70y	625	900	300
	9-13y	420	600	1700
	14-18y	485	700	2800
	19-30y	500	700	3000
	31-50y	500	700	3000
	51-70y	500	700	3000
Females	>70y	500	700	3000
	14-18y	530	750	2800
	19-30y	550	770	3000
Pregnancy	31-50y	550	770	3000
	14-18y	885	1200	2800
	19-30y	900	1300	3000
Lactation	31-50y	900	1300	3000

Function: Required for normal vision, gene expression, reproduction, embryonic development and immune function.

Selected food sources: Liver, dairy products, fish, darkly colored fruits, leafy vegetables.

Adverse effects of excessive consumption: Teratological effects, liver toxicity. Note: From preformed Vitamin A only.

Special considerations: Individuals with high alcohol intake, preexisting liver disease, hyperlipidemia or severe protein malnutrition may be distinctly susceptible to the adverse effects of excess preformed vitamin A intake. β-carotene supplements are advised only to serve as a provitamin A source for individuals at risk of vitamin A deficiency.

Vitamin B1

Member of the vitamin B complex. Known also as thiamin and aneurin. Supplied in supplements and in food fortification as hydrochloride or nitrate. First isolated from rice polishing by Dr. B.C.P. Jansen and Dr. W.F.Donath in 1926.

Vitamin B1 - Thiamin - (mg/d)				
Age		EAR	RDA/AI	UL
Infant	0-6mo	N/A	0.2	ND
	6-12mo	N/A	0.3	ND
Children	1-3y	0.4	0.5	ND
	4-8y	0.5	0.6	ND
Males	9-13y	0.7	0.9	ND
	14-18y	1	1.2	ND
	19-30y	1	1.2	ND
	31-50y	1	1.2	ND
	51-70y	1	1.2	ND
	>70y	1	1.2	ND
Females	9-13y	0.7	0.9	ND
	14-18y	0.9	1	ND
	19-30y	0.9	1.1	ND
	31-50y	0.9	1.1	ND
	51-70y	0.9	1.1	ND
	>70y	0.9	1.1	ND
Pregnancy	14-18y	1.2	1.4	ND
	19-30y	1.2	1.4	ND
	31-50y	1.2	1.4	ND
Lactation	14-18y	1.2	1.4	ND
	19-30y	1.2	1.4	ND
	31-50y	1.2	1.4	ND

Function: Coenzyme in the metabolism of carbohydrates

and branched chain amino acids.

Selected food sources: Enriched, fortified, or whole-grain products; bread and bread products, mixed foods with main ingredient grain, and ready-to eat cereals

Adverse effects of excessive consumption: No adverse effects associated with thiamin from food or supplements have been reported. This does not mean that there is no potential for adverse effects resulting from high intakes. Because data on the adverse effects of thiamin are limited, caution may be warranted.

Special considerations: Persons who may have increased needs for thiamin include those being treated with hemodialysis or peritoneal dialysis, or individuals with malabsorption syndrome.

Vitamin B2

Member of vitamin B complex. Has strong yellow colour, enough to cause high coloured urine, but is harmless. Known as riboflavin, lactoflavin, vitamin G. Isolated from whey by Dr. R Kuhn in 1933, after recognition in yeast by Dr. O. Warburg in 1932.

Riboflavin-B2-(mg/d)				
Age		EAR	RDA/AI	UL
Infant	0-6mo	N/A	0.3	ND
	6-12mo	N/A	0.4	ND
Children	1-3y	0	0.5	ND
	4-8y	0.5	0.6	ND
Males	9-13y	0.8	0.9	ND
	14-18y	1.1	1.3	ND
	19-30y	1.1	1.3	ND
	31-50y	1.1	1.3	ND
	51-70y	1.1	1.3	ND
	>70y	1.1	1.3	ND
Females	9-13y	0.8	0.9	ND
	14-18y	0.9	1	ND
	19-30y	0.9	1.1	ND
	31-50y	0.9	1.1	ND
	51-70y	0.9	1.1	ND
	>70y	0.9	1.1	ND
Pregnancy	14-18y	1.2	1.4	ND
	19-30y	1.2	1.4	ND
	31-50y	1.2	1.4	ND
Lactation	14-18y	1.3	1.6	ND
	19-30y	1.3	1.6	ND
	31-50y	1.3	1.6	ND

Function: Coenzyme in numerous redox reactions.

Selected food sources: Organ meats, milk, bread products and fortified cereals.

Adverse effects of excessive consumption: No adverse effects associated with riboflavin consumption from food or supplements have been reported. This does not mean that there is no potential for adverse effects resulting from high intakes. Because data on the adverse effects of riboflavin are limited, caution may be warranted.

Special considerations: None

Vitamin B3

Water-soluble vitamin, member of vitamin B complex. Known as nicotinic acid, niacinamide, nicotinamide, niacin, vitamin PP or PP factor (pellagra-preventing = PP). Nicotinic acid known since 1867, but rediscovered as a vitamin in 1937 by Dr. C.Elvehjem.

Niacin - B3 - (mg/d)				
Age		EAR	RDA/AI	UL
Infant	0-6mo	N/A	2	ND
	6-12mo	N/A	4	ND
Children	1-3y	5	6	10
	4-8y	6	8	15
Males	9-13y	9	12	20
	14-18y	12	16	30
	19-30y	12	16	35
	31-50y	12	16	35
	51-70y	12	16	35
	>70y	12	16	35
Females	9-13y	9	12	20
	14-18y	11	14	30
	19-30y	11	14	35
	31-50y	11	14	35
	51-70y	11	14	35
	>70y	11	14	35
Pregnancy	14-18y	14	18	30
	19-30y	14	18	35
	31-50y	14	18	35
Lactation	14-18y	13	17	30
	19-30y	13	17	35
	31-50y	13	17	35

Function: Coenzyme or cosubstrate in many biological reduction and oxidation reactions - thus required for energy metabolism.

Selected food sources: Meat, fish, poultry, enriched and wholegrain breads and bread products, fortified ready-to-eat cereals.

Adverse effects of excessive consumption: There is no evidence of adverse effects from the consumption of naturally occurring niacin in foods. Adverse effects from niacin containing supplements may include flushing and gastrointestinal distress. The UL for niacin applies to synthetic forms obtained from supplements, fortified foods, or a combination of the two.

Special considerations: Extra niacin may be required by persons treated with hemodialysis or peritoneal dialysis, or those with malabsorption syndrome.

Vitamin B5

Pantothenic acid, from panthos meaning everywhere in Greek. Water soluble vitamin, member of vitamin B complex. Usually presented in oral supplements as calcium pantothenate, in cosmetics and toiletries as dexpanthenol and pantothenol. Known as vitamin B5, chick antidermatitis factor, and anti-stress vitamin. Isolated from rice husks by Dr. R.J.Williams in 1939. Naturally as D-pantothenic acid.

Pantothenic acid - B5 - (µg/d)				
Age		EAR	RDA/AI	UL
Infant	0-6mo	N/A	1.7	ND
	6-12mo	N/A	1.8	ND
Children	1-3y	N/A	2	ND
	4-8y	N/A	3	ND
Males	9-13y	N/A	4	ND
	14-18y	N/A	5	ND
	19-30y	N/A	5	ND
	31-50y	N/A	5	ND
	51-70y	N/A	5	ND
	>70y	N/A	5	ND
Females	9-13y	N/A	4	ND
	14-18y	N/A	5	ND
	19-30y	N/A	5	ND
	31-50y	N/A	5	ND
	51-70y	N/A	5	ND
	>70y	N/A	5	ND
Pregnancy	14-18y	N/A	6	ND
	19-30y	N/A	6	ND
	31-50y	N/A	6	ND
Lactation	14-18y	N/A	7	ND
	19-30y	N/A	7	ND
	31-50y	N/A	7	ND

Function: Coenzyme in fatty acid metabolism.

Selected food sources: Chicken, beef, potatoes, oats, cereals, tomato products, liver, kidney, yeast, egg yolk, broccoli, whole grains.

Adverse effects of excessive consumption: No adverse effects associated with pantothenic acid from food or supplements have been reported. This does not mean that there is no potential for adverse effects resulting from high intakes. Because data on the adverse effects of pantothenic acid are limited, caution may be warranted.

Special considerations: None

Vitamin B6

Water soluble vitamin, member of vitamin B complex. Known as pyridoxine, pyridoxal and pyridoxamine. Present in supplements as hydroxychloride and phosphate. Antidepressant vitamin. Isolated from liver by Pr. Paul Gyorgy in 1934.

Vitamin B6 (mg/d)				
Age		EAR	RDA/AI	UL
Infant	0-6mo	N/A	0.1	ND
	6-12mo	N/A	0.3	ND
Children	1-3y	0.4	0.5	30
	4-8y	0.5	0.6	40
Males	9-13y	0.8	1	60
	14-18y	1.1	1.3	80
	19-30y	1.1	1.3	100
	31-50y	1.1	1.3	100
	51-70y	1.4	1.7	100
	>70y	1.4	1.7	100
Females	9-13y	0.8	1	60
	14-18y	1	1.2	80
	19-30y	1.1	1.3	100
	31-50y	1.1	1.3	100
	51-70y	1.3	1.5	100
	>70y	1.3	1.5	100
Pregnancy	14-18y	1.6	1.9	80
	19-30y	1.6	1.9	100
	31-50y	1.6	1.9	100
Lactation	14-18y	1.7	2	80
	19-30y	1.7	2	100
	31-50y	1.7	2	100

Function: Coenzyme in the metabolism of amino acids, glycogen and sphingoid bases

Selected food sources: Fortified cereals, organ meats, fortified soy-based meat substitutes.

Adverse effects of excessive consumption: No adverse effects associated with Vitamin B6 from food have been reported. This does not mean that there is no potential for adverse effects resulting from high intakes. Because data on the adverse effects of Vitamin B6 are limited, caution may be warranted. Sensory neuropathy has occurred from high intakes of supplemental forms.

Special considerations: None

Vitamin B9

Water soluble vitamin, member of vitamin B complex, known as folic acid, vitamin Bc, vitamin M, pteroyl glutamic acid, PGA, liver lactobacillus case factor, folacin, anti-anaemia vitamin. Isolated in 1939 from liver, in 1945 Dr. Tom Spies demonstrated it cured anemia of pregnancy.

Folate - B9 (µg/d)				
Age		EAR	RDA/AI	UL
Infant	0-6mo	N/A	65	ND
	6-12mo	N/A	80	ND
Children	1-3y	120	150	300
	4-8y	160	200	400
Males	9-13y	250	300	600
	14-18y	330	400	800
	19-30y	320	400	1000
	31-50y	320	400	1000
	51-70y	320	400	1000
	>70y	320	400	1000
Females	9-13y	250	300	600
	14-18y	330	400	800
	19-30y	320	400	1000
	31-50y	320	400	1000
	51-70y	320	400	1000
	>70y	320	400	1000
Pregnancy	14-18y	520	600	800
	19-30y	520	600	1000
	31-50y	520	600	1000
Lactation	14-18y	450	500	800
	19-30y	450	500	1000
	31-50y	450	500	1000

Function: Coenzyme in the metabolism of nucleic and

amino acids; prevents megaloblastic anemia.

Selected food sources: Enriched cereal grains, dark leafy vegetables, enriched and whole-grain breads and bread products, fortified ready-to-eat cereals.

Adverse effects of excessive consumption: Masks neurological complication in people with vitamin B12 deficiency. No adverse effects associated with folate from food or supplements have been reported. This does not mean that there is no potential for adverse effects resulting from high intakes. Because data on the adverse effects of folate are limited, caution may be warranted. The UL for folate applies to synthetic forms obtained from supplements and/or fortified foods.

Special considerations: In view of evidence linking folate intake with neural tube defects in the fetus, it is recommended that all women capable of becoming pregnant consume 400 µg from supplements or fortified foods in addition to intake of food folate from a varied diet. It is assumed that women will continue consuming 400 µg from supplements or fortified food until their pregnancy is confirmed and they enter prenatal care, which ordinarily occurs after the end of the periconceptional period - the critical time for formation of the neural tube.

Vitamin B12

Contains cobalt, known as cobalamin. Water soluble vitamin, member of vitamin B complex. Synonymous with anti-pernicious anemia vitamin, cyano-cobalamin, hydroxicobalamin, aquacobalamin, LLD factor, extrinsic vitamin, animal protein factor. Deep red crystalline substance. Last true vitamin to be discovered, isolated from liver in 1848 by Pr. E.L.Smith in UK in the same time with Dr. K.Folkers in US. Now is obtained by deep fermentation.

B12 (µg/d)				
Age		EAR	RDA/AI	UL
Infant	0-6mo	N/A	0.4	
	6-12mo	N/A	0.5	
Children	1-3y	0.7	0.9	
	4-8y	1	1.2	
Males	9-13y	1.5	1.8	
	14-18y	2	2.4	
	19-30y	2	2.4	
	31-50y	2	2.4	
	51-70y	2	2.4	
	>70y	2	2.4	
Females	9-13y	1.5	1.8	
	14-18y	2	2.4	
	19-30y	2	2.4	
	31-50y	2	2.4	
	51-70y	2	2.4	
	>70y	2	2.4	
Pregnancy	14-18y	2.2	2.6	
	19-30y	2.2	2.6	
	31-50y	2.2	2.6	
Lactation	14-18y	2.4	2.8	
	19-30y	2.4	2.8	
	31-50y	2.4	2.8	

Function: Coenzyme in nucleic acid metabolism; prevents megaloblastic anemia.

Selected food sources: Fortified cereals, meat, fish, poultry.

Adverse effects of excessive consumption: No adverse effects have been associated with the consumption of the amounts of vitamin B12 normally found in foods or supplements. This does not mean that there is no potential for adverse effects resulting from high intakes. Because data on the adverse effects of vitamin B12 are limited, caution may be warranted.

Special considerations: Because 10 to 30 percent of older people may malabsorb food bound vitamin B12, it is advisable for those older than 50 years to meet their RDA mainly by consuming foods fortified with vitamin B12 or a supplement containing vitamin B12.

Biotin

Water soluble vitamin, member of vitamin B complex. Known as vitamin H, bios II, coenzyme R. Isolated from liver by Dr. Paul Gyorgy in 1941. Natural form is D-biotin.

Biotin (µg/d)				
Age		EAR	RDA/AI	UL
	0-6mo	N/A	5	ND
Infant	6-12mo	N/A	6	ND
	1-3y	N/A	8	ND
Children	4-8y	N/A	12	ND
	9-13y	N/A	20	ND
	14-18y	N/A	25	ND
	19-30y	N/A	30	ND
	31-50y	N/A	30	ND
	51-70y	N/A	30	ND
Males	>70y	N/A	30	ND
	9-13y	N/A	20	ND
	14-18y	N/A	25	ND
	19-30y	N/A	30	ND
	31-50y	N/A	30	ND
	51-70y	N/A	30	ND
Females	>70y	N/A	30	ND
	14-18y	N/A	30	ND
	19-30y	N/A	30	ND
Pregnancy	31-50y	N/A	30	ND
	14-18y	N/A	35	ND
	19-30y	N/A	35	ND
Lactation	31-50y	N/A	35	ND

Function: Coenzyme in synthesis of fat, glycogen, and amino acids

Selected food sources: Liver and smaller amounts in fruits

George C. Mihalache

and meats.

Adverse effects of excessive consumption: No adverse effects of biotin in humans or animals were found. This does not mean that there is no potential for adverse effects resulting from high intakes. Because data on the adverse effects of biotin are limited, caution may be warranted.

Special considerations: None

34

Vitamin C

Water soluble vitamin. Known also as L-ascorbic acid, anti-scorbutic acid, hexuronic acid, cevitaminic acid, ascorbyl palmitate, ascorbyl nicotinate. White, crystalline powder, isolated from fruits, paprika and adrenal glands by Dr. A.Szent-Gyorgy in 1922.

Vitamin C (mg/d)		EAR	RDA/AI	UL
Age		EAR	RDA/AI	UL
	0-6mo	N/A	40*	ND
Infant	6-12mo	N/A	50*	NDD
	1-3y	13	15	400
Children	4-8y	22	25	650
	9-13y	39	45	1200
	14-18y	63	75	1800
	19-30y	75	90	2000
	31-50y	75	90	2000
	51-70y	75	90	2000
Males	>70y	75	90	2000
	9-13y	39	45	1200
	14-18y	56	65	1800
	19-30y	60	75	2000
	31-50y	60	75	2000
	51-70y	60	75	2000
Females	>70y	60	75	2000
	14-18y	66	80	1800
	19-30y	70	85	2000
Pregnancy	31-50y	70	85	2000
	14-18y	96	115	2000
	19-30y	100	120	2000
Lactation	31-50y	100	120	2000

Function: Cofactor for reactions requiring reduced copper or iron metalloenzyme and as a protective antioxidant

Selected food sources: Citrus fruits, tomatoes, tomato juice, potatoes, Bruxelles sprouts, cauliflower, broccoli, strawberries, cabbage and spinach.

Adverse effects of excessive consumption: Gastrointestinal disturbances, kidney stones, excess iron absorption.

Special considerations: Individuals who smoke require an additional 35 mg/d of vitamin C over that needed by nonsmokers. Nonsmokers regularly exposed to tobacco smoke are encouraged to ensure they meet the RDA for vitamin C.

Vitamin D

Fat soluble vitamin, found as cholecalciferol – D3, as animal origin, or ergocalciferol – D2, produced by action of light on yeast. Isolated in 1930 from liver oil by Dr. E. Mallanby. Sunshine vitamin.

Vitamin D (µg/d)				
Age		EAR	RDA/AI	UL
Infant	0-6mo	N/A	10	25
	6-12mo	N/A	10	38
Children	1-3y	10	15	63
	4-8y	10	15	75
Males	9-13y	10	15	100
	14-18y	10	15	100
	19-30y	10	15	100
	31-50y	10	15	100
	51-70y	10	15	100
	>70y	10	20	100
Females	9-13y	10	15	100
	14-18y	10	15	100
	19-30y	10	15	100
	31-50y	10	15	100
	51-70y	10	15	100
	>70y	10	20	100
Pregnancy	14-18y	10	15	100
	19-30y	10	15	100
	31-50y	10	15	100
Lactation	14-18y	10	15	100
	19-30y	10	15	100
	31-50y	10	15	100

Function: Maintain serum calcium and phosphorus concentrations, and in turn, bone health.

Selected food sources: Fish liver oils, flesh of fatty fish, egg yolk, fortified dairy products and fortified cereals.

Adverse effects of excessive consumption: Hypercalcemia which can lead to decreased renal function and hypercalciuria, kidney failure, cardiovascular system failure, and calcification of soft tissues.

Special considerations: None

Vitamin E

Tocopherol from tokos – birth and phero – bear. Fat soluble vitamin. Known as d-alpha tocopherol (natural) and found in supplements as d-alpha tocopheryl acetate or d-alpha tocopheryl succinate, sometimes as synthetic dl-alpha tocopherol.

Vitamin E (mg/d)				
Age		EAR	RDA/AI	UL
Infant	0-6mo	N/A	4	ND
	6-12mo	N/A	5	ND
Children	1-3y	5	6	200
	4-8y	6	7	300
Males	9-13y	9	11	600
	14-18y	12	15	800
	19-30y	12	15	1000
	31-50y	12	15	1000
	51-70y	12	15	1000
	>70y	12	15	1000
Females	9-13y	9	11	600
	14-18y	12	15	800
	19-30y	12	15	1000
	31-50y	12	15	1000
	51-70y	12	15	1000
	>70y	12	15	100
Pregnancy	14-18y	12	15	800
	19-30y	12	15	1000
	31-50y	12	15	1000
Lactation	14-18y	16	19	800
	19-30y	16	19	1000
	31-50y	16	19	1000

Function: A metabolic function has not yet been identified.

Vitamin E's major function appears to be as a nonspecific chain-breaking antioxidant.

Selected food sources: Vegetable oils, unprocessed cereal grains, nuts, fruits, vegetables, meats.

Adverse effects of excessive consumption: There is no evidence of adverse effects from the consumption of vitamin E naturally occurring in foods. Adverse effects from vitamin E containing supplements may include hemorrhagic toxicity. The UL for vitamin E applies to any form of α-tocopherol obtained from supplements, fortified foods, or a combination of the two.

Special considerations: Patients on anticoagulant therapy should be monitored when taking vitamin E supplements.

Vitamin K

Fat soluble vitamin, derived from koagulation (Danish). Known as vitamin K, phytomenadione, phyloquinone, phytylmenadione, anti-haemorrhagic vitamin. Produced by intestinal bacteria as K2, Synthetic vitamin is K3, known as menadione and menaphtone. K1 was isolated from alfalfa by Dr. H.Dam in 1935; K2 was isolated from decayed fishmeal in 1939.

Vitamin K (µg/d)				
Age		EAR	AI	UL
Infant	0-6mo	N/A	2	ND
	6-12mo	N/A	2.5	ND
Children	1-3y	N/A	30	ND
	4-8y	N/A	55	ND
Males	9-13y	N/A	60	ND
	14-18y	N/A	75	ND
	19-30y	N/A	120	ND
	31-50y	N/A	120	ND
	51-70y	N/A	120	ND
	>70y	N/A	120	ND
Females	9-13y	N/A	60	ND
	14-18y	N/A	75	ND
	19-30y	N/A	90	ND
	31-50y	N/A	90	ND
	51-70y	N/A	90	ND
	>70y	N/A	90	ND
Pregnancy	14-18y	N/A	75	ND
	19-30y	N/A	90	ND
	31-50y	N/A	90	ND
Lactation	14-18y	N/A	75	ND
	19-30y	N/A	90	ND
	31-50y	N/A	90	ND

Function: Coenzyme during the synthesis of many proteins involved in blood clotting and bone metabolism.

Selected food sources: Green vegetables (collards, spinach, salad greens, broccoli), Brussels sprouts, cabbage, plant oils and margarine.

Adverse effects of excessive consumption: No adverse effects associated with vitamin K consumption from food or supplements have been reported in humans or animals. This does not mean that there is no potential for adverse effects resulting from high intakes. Because data on the adverse effects of vitamin K are limited, caution may be warranted.

Special considerations: Patients on anticoagulant therapy should monitor vitamin K intake.

George C. Mihalache

Chapter 2

MINERALS

George C. Mihalache

2. MINERALS

INTRODUCTION

The body needs many minerals; these are called essential minerals. Essential minerals are sometimes divided up into **major minerals** (macro-minerals) and **trace minerals** (micro-minerals). These two groups of minerals are equally important, but **trace minerals** are needed in smaller amounts than major minerals. The amounts needed in the body are not an indication of their importance. A balanced diet usually provides all of the essential minerals. Literally, they mean "mined from the earth". They are divided in metallic elements, present in high quantities in the body and diet where daily intakes are greater than 100mg (calcium, magnesium, potassium); non-metallic elements, abundant in the earth, body and diet, where daily intakes are greater than 100mg (carbon, phosphorus, sulphur); metallic elements, present in very small amounts in the body and diet, that are essential for health (chromium, copper, iron); non-metallic elements, present in very small amounts in the body and diet, that are essential for health (fluorine, iodine, selenium). Any essential element not found in group 1 or 2 is classed as a **trace mineral** or trace element.

Calcium

Chemical symbol Ca, atomic weight 40.08. A metallic macro-element present in skeleton and teeth (1100g) with the remaining 10g in nerves, muscles and blood. Calcium in the blood is essential in blood clotting. In the nerves and muscles for nerve impulse transmission and muscular function.

Calcium (mg/d)				
Age		EAR	RDA/AI	UL
Infant	0-6mo	N/A	200	1000
	6-12mo	N/A	260	1500
Children	1-3y	500	700	2500
	4-8y	800	1000	2500
Males	9-13y	1100	1300	3000
	14-18y	1100	1300	3000
	19-30y	800	1000	2500
	31-50y	800	1000	2500
	51-70y	800	1000	2000
	>70y	1000	1000	2500
Females	9-13y	1100	1300	3000
	14-18y	1100	1300	3000
	19-30y	800	1000	2500
	31-50y	800	1000	2000
	51-70y	1000	1200	2000
	>70y	1000	1000	2000
Pregnancy	14-18y	1000	1300	3000
	19-30y	800	1300	3000
	31-50y	800	1300	3000
Lactation	14-18y	1000	1000	2500
	19-30y	800	1000	2500
	31-50y	800	1000	2500

Function: Essential role in blood clotting, muscle

contraction, nerve transmission, and bone and tooth formation.

Selected food sources: Milk, cheese, yogurt, corn tortillas, calcium-set tofu, Chinese cabbage, kale, broccoli, as well as other fortified foods and beverages.

Adverse effects of excessive consumption: Kidney stones, hypercalcemia, hypercalciuria, prostate cancer, constipation, soft, tissue calcification

Special considerations: None

Chromium

Chemical symbol Cr, atomic weight 52.0, exists in many forms, but trivalent chromium is the only one that can be used by the body. An essential trace element for animals and man.

Chromium (mg/d)				
Age		EAR	RDA/AI	UL
Infant	0-6mo	N/A	0.2	ND
	6-12mo	N/A	5.5	ND
Children	1-3y	N/A	11	ND
	4-8y	N/A	15	ND
Males	9-13y	N/A	25	ND
	14-18y	N/A	35	ND
	19-30y	N/A	35	ND
	31-50y	N/A	35	ND
	51-70y	N/A	30	ND
	>70y	N/A	30	ND
Females	9-13y	N/A	21	ND
	14-18y	N/A	24	ND
	19-30y	N/A	25	ND
	31-50y	N/A	25	ND
	51-70y	N/A	20	ND
	>70y	N/A	20	ND
Pregnancy	14-18y	N/A	29	ND
	19-30y	N/A	30	ND
	31-50y	N/A	30	ND
Lactation	14-18y	N/A	44	ND
	19-30y	N/A	45	ND
	31-50y	N/A	45	ND

Function: Helps to maintain normal blood glucose levels.

Selected food sources: Some cereals, meats, poultry, fish and beer.

Adverse effects of excessive consumption: Chronic renal

failure.
Special considerations: None

Chloride

Chemical symbol Cl, atomic weight 35.5, abundance in igneous rock is 0.031 % by weight, in sea water 1.9% by weight, primarily as sodium chloride (sea salt). An essential mineral form of chlorine in plants, animals and man.

Chloride (g/d)				
Age		EAR	RDA/AI	UL
	0-6mo	N/A	0.18	ND
Infant	6-12mo	N/A	0.57	ND
	1-3y	N/A	1.5	2.3
Children	4-8y	N/A	1.9	2.9
	9-13y	N/A	2.3	3.4
	14-18y	N/A	2.3	3.6
	19-30y	N/A	2.3	3.6
	31-50y	N/A	2.3	3.6
	51-70y	N/A	2	3.6
Males	>70y	N/A	1.8	3.6
	9-13y	N/A	2.3	3.4
	14-18y	N/A	2.3	3.6
	19-30y	N/A	2.3	3.6
	31-50y	N/A	2.3	3.6
	51-70y	N/A	2	3.6
Females	>70y	N/A	1.8	3.6
	14-18y	N/A	2.3	3.6
	19-30y	N/A	2.3	3.6
Pregnancy	31-50y	N/A	2.3	3.6
	14-18y	N/A	2.3	3.6
	19-30y	N/A	2.3	3.6
Lactation	31-50y	N/A	2.3	3.6

Function: act as the main anion to sodium and potassium cations in maintenance of body water levels and neutrality, provide chloride for the production of hydrochloric acid by the stomach.

Selected food sources: food rich in sodium and potassium is rich in chloride.

Adverse effects of excessive consumption: same as for sodium and potassium.

Special considerations: None

Copper

Chemical symbol Cu, from the Latin cuprum, atomic weight 63.5. An essential trace element for man, animals and many plants.

Copper (µg/d)				
Age		EAR	RDA/AI	UL
	0-6mo	N/A	200	ND
Infant	6-12mo	N/A	220	ND
	1-3y	260	340	1000
Children	4-8y	340	440	3000
	9-13y	540	700	5000
	14-18y	685	890	8000
	19-30y	700	900	10000
	31-50y	700	900	10000
	51-70y	700	900	10000
Males	>70y	700	900	10000
	9-13y	540	700	5000
	14-18y	685	890	8000
	19-30y	700	900	10000
	31-50y	700	900	10000
	51-70y	700	900	10000
Females	>70y	700	900	10000
	14-18y	785	1000	8000
	19-30y	800	1000	10000
Pregnancy	31-50y	800	1000	10000
	14-18y	985	1300	8000
	19-30y	1000	1300	10000
Lactation	31-50y	1000	1300	10000

Function: Component of enzymes in iron metabolism.
Selected food sources: Organ meats, seafood, nuts, seeds, wheat bran cereals, whole grain products, cocoa

products.

Adverse effects of excessive consumption: Gastrointestinal distress, liver damage.

Special considerations: Individuals with Wilson's disease, Indian childhood cirrhosis and idiopathic copper toxicosis may be at an increased risk of adverse effects from excess copper intake.

Iodine

Chemical symbol I, atomic weight 126.9. An essential trace element for animals and man.

Iodine (µg/d)				
Age		EAR	RDA/AI	UL
Infant	0-6mo	N/A	110	ND
	6-12mo	N/A	130	ND
Children	1-3y	65	90	200
	4-8y	65	90	300
Males	9-13y	73	120	600
	14-18y	95	150	900
	19-30y	95	150	1100
	31-50y	95	150	1100
	51-70y	95	150	1100
	>70y	95	150	1100
Females	9-13y	73	120	600
	14-18y	95	150	900
	19-30y	95	150	1100
	31-50y	95	150	1100
	51-70y	95	150	1100
	>70y	95	150	1100
Pregnancy	14-18y	160	220	900
	19-30y	160	220	1100
	31-50y	160	220	1100
Lactation	14-18y	209	290	900
	19-30y	209	290	1100
	31-50y	209	290	1100

Function: Component of the thyroid hormones; and prevents goiter and cretinism.

Selected food sources: Marine origin, processed foods, iodized salt.

Adverse effects of excessive consumption: Elevated

thyroid stimulating hormone (TSH) concentration.

Special considerations: Individuals with autoimmune thyroid disease, previous iodine deficiency, or nodular goiter are distinctly susceptible to the adverse effect of excess iodine intake. Therefore, individuals with these conditions may not be protected by the UL for iodine intake for the general population.

Iron

Chemical symbol Fe, from Latin ferum, atomic weight 55.95, exists as ferrous acid and ferric iron. Essential trace mineral that is present in the body to the extent of 3.5 to 4.5g. Approx. 66% is present as hemoglobin, the red oxygen-carrying pigment of blood. The remaining 33% is stored in the liver, spleen, bone marrow and muscles (where is present as myoglobin, that acts as oxygen reservoir within the muscle fiber). In the organs and in the blood plasma iron exists as protein complex.

Iron (mg/d)				
Age		EAR	RDA/AI	UL
	0-6mo	N/A	0.27	40
Infant	6-12mo	6.9	11	40
	1-3y	3	7	40
Children	4-8y	4.1	10	40
	9-13y	5.9	8	40
	14-18y	7.7	11	45
	19-30y	6	8	45
	31-50y	6	8	45
	51-70y	6	8	45
Males	>70y	6	8	45
	9-13y	5.7	8	40
	14-18y	7.9	15	45
	19-30y	8.1	18	45
	31-50y	8.1	18	45
	51-70y	5	8	45
Females	>70y	5	8	45
	14-18y	23	27	45
	19-30y	22	27	45
Pregnancy	31-50y	22	27	45
	14-18y	7	10	45
	19-30y	6.5	9	45
Lactation	31-50y	6.5	9	45

Function: Component of hemoglobin and numerous enzymes; prevents microcytic hypochromic anemia.

Selected food sources: Fruits, vegetables and fortified bread and grain products such as cereal (nonheme iron sources), meat and poultry (heme iron sources).

Adverse effects of excessive consumption: Gastrointestinal distress.

Special considerations: Non-heme iron absorption is lower for those consuming vegetarian diets than for those eating non-vegetarian diets. Therefore, it has been suggested that the iron requirement for those consuming a vegetarian diet is approximately 2-fold greater than for those consuming a non-vegetarian diet. Recommended intake assumes 75% of iron is from heme iron sources.

Manganese

Chemical symbol Mn, atomic weight 54.9. An essential trace element for human beings.

Manganese (mg/d)				
Age		EAR	RDA/AI	UL
	0-6mo	N/A	0.003	ND
Infant	6-12mo	N/A	0.6	ND
	1-3y	N/A	1.2	2
Children	4-8y	N/A	1.5	3
	9-13y	N/A	1.9	6
	14-18y	N/A	2.2	9
	19-30y	N/A	2.3	11
	31-50y	N/A	2.3	11
	51-70y	N/A	2.3	11
Males	>70y	N/A	2.3	11
	9-13y	N/A	1.6	6
	14-18y	N/A	1.6	9
	19-30y	N/A	1.8	11
	31-50y	N/A	1.8	11
	51-70y	N/A	1.8	11
Females	>70y	N/A	1.8	11
	14-18y	N/A	2	9
	19-30y	N/A	2	11
Pregnancy	31-50y	N/A	2	11
	14-18y	N/A	2.6	9
	19-30y	N/A	2.6	11
Lactation	31-50y	N/A	2.6	11

Function: Involved in the formation of bone, as well as in enzymes involved in amino acid, cholesterol, and carbohydrate metabolism.

Selected food sources: Nuts, legumes, tea, and whole grains.

Adverse effects of excessive consumption: Elevated blood concentration and neurotoxicity

Special considerations: Because manganese in drinking water and supplements may be more bioavailable than manganese from food, caution should be taken when using manganese supplements especially among those persons already consuming large amounts of manganese from diets high in plant products. In addition, individuals with liver disease may be distinctly susceptible to the adverse effects of excess manganese intake.

Magnesium

Chemical symbol Mg, atomic weight 24.31, name derived from the Greek city of Magnesia, where there are large deposits of magnesium carbonate. Body contains about 25g of magnesium, 50% of it found in the bones. The rest is distributed amongst organs, nerves and blood.

Magnesium (mg/d)				
Age		EAR	RDA/AI	UL
	0-6mo	N/A	30	ND
Infant	6-12mo	N/A	75	ND
	1-3y	65	80	65
Children	4-8y	110	130	110
	9-13y	200	240	350
	14-18y	340	410	350
	19-30y	330	400	350
	31-50y	350	420	350
	51-70y	350	420	350
Males	>70y	350	420	350
	9-13y	200	240	350
	14-18y	300	360	350
	19-30y	255	310	350
	31-50y	265	320	350
	51-70y	265	320	350
Females	>70y	265	320	350
	14-18y	335	400	350
	19-30y	290	350	350
Pregnancy	31-50y	300	360	350
	14-18y	300	360	350
	19-30y	255	310	350
Lactation	31-50y	265	320	350

Function: Cofactor for enzyme systems.
Selected food sources: Green leafy vegetables,

unpolished grains, nuts, meat, starches, milk.

Adverse effects of excessive consumption: There is no evidence of adverse effects from the consumption of naturally occurring magnesium in foods. Adverse effects from magnesium containing supplements may include osmotic diarrhea. The UL for magnesium represents intake from a pharmacological agent only and does not include intake from food and water.

Special considerations: None

Molybdenum

Chemical symbol Mo, atomic weight 95.9, Essential in soil and plants for processes utilizing nitrogen from the air. Essential trace element for animals and man.

Molybdenum (µg/d)				
Age		EAR	RDA/AI	UL
Infant	0-6mo	N/A	2	ND
	6-12mo	N/A	3	ND
Children	1-3y	13	17	300
	4-8y	17	22	600
Males	9-13y	26	34	1100
	14-18y	33	43	1700
	19-30y	34	45	2000
	31-50y	34	45	2000
	51-70y	34	45	2000
	>70y	34	45	2000
Females	9-13y	26	34	1100
	14-18y	33	43	1700
	19-30y	34	45	2000
	31-50y	34	45	2000
	51-70y	34	45	2000
	>70y	34	45	2000
Pregnancy	14-18y	40	50	1700
	19-30y	40	50	2000
	31-50y	40	50	2000
Lactation	14-18y	35	50	1700
	19-30y	36	50	2000
	31-50y	36	50	2000

Function: Cofactor for enzymes involved in catabolism of sulfur amino acids, purines and pyridines.

Selected food sources: Legumes, grain products and nuts.

Adverse effects of excessive consumption: Reproductive effects as observed in animal studies.

Special considerations: Individuals who are deficient in dietary copper intake or have some dysfunction in copper metabolism that makes them copper deficient could be at increased risk of molybdenum toxicity.

Potassium

Chemical symbol K, from Latin kalium, atomic weight 39, alkali metal that is found mainly as sylvite (potassium chloride), in the aliminosilicates orthoclase and microcline, or as carnallite. Occurrence in earth's crust is 2.59%. The body potassium content of an average person is about 150g, of this only 3.2g is present in the extracellular fluid. The remaining 147g can be found inside body cells and of this, 80% is present in skeletal muscles. The quantity in the skeleton is negligible.

Potassium (g/d)				
Age		EAR	RDA/AI	UL
Infant	0-6mo	N/A	0.4	NONE
	6-12mo	N/A	0.7	NONE
Children	1-3y	N/A	3	NONE
	4-8y	N/A	3.8	NONE
Males	9-13y	N/A	4.5	NONE
	14-18y	N/A	4.7	NONE
	19-30y	N/A	4.7	NONE
	31-50y	N/A	4.7	NONE
	51-70y	N/A	4.7	NONE
	>70y	N/A	4.7	NONE
Females	9-13y	N/A	4.5	NONE
	14-18y	N/A	4.7	NONE
	19-30y	N/A	4.7	NONE
	31-50y	N/A	4.7	NONE
	51-70y	N/A	4.7	NONE
	>70y	N/A	4.7	NONE
Pregnancy	14-18y	N/A	4.7	NONE
	19-30y	N/A	4.7	NONE
	31-50y	N/A	4.7	NONE
Lactation	14-18y	N/A	4.7	NONE
	19-30y	N/A	5.1	NONE
	31-50y	N/A	5.1	NONE

Function: maintaining a normal balance of water within body cells as the major positively-charged ion within these cells, activator in a number of enzymes, particularly those concerned with energy production, stabilize the internal structure of body cells, assisting specialized cell particles to synthetize proteins, nerve impulse transmission, increasing the excitability of heart and skeletal muscle to make them more receptive to nerve impulses, preserving the acid-alkali balance in the body, stimulating the normal movements in the intestinal tract.

Selected food sources: dried fruits, soy flour, molasses, wheat bran, raw salad, chipped potato, nuts

Adverse effects of excessive consumption: Kidney failure, insufficient production of adrenal gland hormones.

Special considerations: None

Phosphorus

Chemical symbol P, atomic weight 30.9, present in the body (combined with oxygen) as phosphates, it is a constituent of all plant and animal cell.

Phosphorus (mg/d)				
Age		EAR	RDA/AI	UL
Infant	0-6mo	N/A	100	ND
	6-12mo	N/A	275	ND
Children	1-3y	380	460	3000
	4-8y	405	500	3000
Males	9-13y	1055	1250	4000
	14-18y	1055	1250	4000
	19-30y	580	700	4000
	31-50y	580	700	4000
	51-70y	580	700	4000
	>70y	580	700	3000
Females	9-13y	1055	1250	4000
	14-18y	1055	1250	4000
	19-30y	580	700	4000
	31-50y	580	700	4000
	51-70y	580	700	4000
	>70y	580	700	3000
Pregnancy	14-18y	1055	1250	3500
	19-30y	580	700	3500
	31-50y	580	700	3500
Lactation	14-18y	1055	1250	4000
	19-30y	580	700	4000
	31-50y	580	700	4000

Function: Maintenance of pH, storage and transfer of energy and nucleotide synthesis.
Selected food sources: Milk, yogurt, ice cream, cheese,

peas, meat, eggs, some cereals and breads.

Adverse effects of excessive consumption: Metastatic calcification, skeletal porosity, interference with calcium absorption.

Special considerations: Athletes and others with high energy expenditure frequently consume amounts from food greater than the UL without apparent effect. A problem can arise from excessive intakes of phosphates from soft drinks, processed foods and fast foods.

Selenium

Chemical symbol Se, atomic weight 79.0, name derived from the moon goddess Selene. An essential trace mineral in animals and man.

Selenium - (µg/d)				
Age		EAR	RDA/AI	UL
	0-6mo	N/A	15	45
Infant	6-12mo	N/A	20	60
	1-3y	17	20	90
Children	4-8y	23	30	150
	9-13y	35	40	280
	14-18y	45	55	400
	19-30y	45	55	400
	31-50y	45	55	400
	51-70y	45	55	400
Males	>70y	45	55	400
	9-13y	35	40	280
	14-18y	45	55	400
	19-30y	45	55	400
	31-50y	45	55	400
	51-70y	45	55	400
Females	>70y	45	55	400
	14-18y	49	60	400
	19-30y	49	60	400
Pregnancy	31-50y	49	60	400
	14-18y	59	70	400
	19-30y	59	70	400
Lactation	31-50y	59	70	400

Function: Defense against oxidative stress and regulation of thyroid hormone action, and the reduction and oxidation status of vitamin C and other molecules.
Selected food sources: Organ meats, seafood, plants

(depending on soil selenium content).

Adverse effects of excessive consumption: Hair and nail brittleness and loss.

Special considerations: None

Sodium

Chemical symbol Na, from Latin natrium, atomic weight 23.0. An alkali metal that occurs naturally as sodium chloride, sodium bromide, sodium silicates and sodium carbonates. Abundance in earth's crust is 2.8%. Adult body content of sodium in a healthy individual is about 92g, equivalent to 234g of sodium chloride. More than 50% is in the extracellular fluids, 34.5g in the bones and less than 11.5g is retained intracellular.

Sodium (g/d)				
Age		EAR	RDA/AI	UL
Infant	0-6mo	N/A	0.12	ND
	6-12mo	N/A	0.37	ND
Children	1-3y	N/A	1	1.5
	4-8y	N/A	1.2	1.9
Males	9-13y	N/A	1.5	2.2
	14-18y	N/A	1.5	2.3
	19-30y	N/A	1.5	2.3
	31-50y	N/A	1.5	2.3
	51-70y	N/A	1.3	2.3
	>70y	N/A	1.2	2.3
Females	9-13y	N/A	1.5	2.2
	14-18y	N/A	1.5	2.3
	19-30y	N/A	1.5	2.3
	31-50y	N/A	1.5	2.3
	51-70y	N/A	1.3	2.3
	>70y	N/A	1.2	2.3
Pregnancy	14-18y	N/A	1.5	2.3
	19-30y	N/A	1.5	2.3
	31-50y	N/A	1.5	2.3
Lactation	14-18y	N/A	1.5	2.3
	19-30y	N/A	1.5	2.3
	31-50y	N/A	1.5	2.3

Function: maintaining a normal balance of water between body cells and the surrounding fluids, nerve impulse transmission, muscle contraction (including heart), preserving acid-alkali balance in the body, constituent of ATPase, the enzyme responsible for splitting adenosine triphosphate in the production of energy, active transport of amino acids and glucose into body cells.

Selected food sources: yeast extract, bacon, smoked fish, salami, sauces, cornflakes, cheese, salted butter.

Adverse effects of excessive consumption: high blood pressure, enlarged heart, enlarged kidney leading to nephritis

Special considerations: Baby's food should not have any salt, as too much salt in a baby's diet can lead to high blood pressure and even death.

Zinc

Chemical symbol Zn, atomic weight 65.4, essential trace mineral for plants, animals and human beings.

Zinc (mg/d)				
Age		EAR	RDA/AI	UL
	0-6mo	N/A	2	4
Infant	6-12mo	2.5	3	5
	1-3y	2.5	3	7
Children	4-8y	4	5	12
	9-13y	7	8	23
	14-18y	8.5	11	34
	19-30y	9.4	11	40
	31-50y	9.4	11	40
	51-70y	9.4	11	40
Males	>70y	9.4	11	40
	9-13y	7	8	23
	14-18y	7.3	9	34
	19-30y	6.8	8	40
	31-50y	6.8	8	40
	51-70y	6.8	8	40
Females	>70y	6.8	8	40
	14-18y	10.5	12	34
	19-30y	9.5	11	40
Pregnancy	31-50y	9.5	11	40
	14-18y	10.9	13	34
	19-30y	10.4	12	40
Lactation	31-50y	10.4	12	40

Function: Component of multiple enzymes and proteins; involved in the regulation of gene expression.

Selected food sources: Fortified cereals, red meats, certain seafood.

Adverse effects of excessive consumption: Reduced copper status.

Special considerations: Zinc absorption is lower for those consuming vegetarian diets than for those eating non-vegetarian diets. Therefore, it has been suggested that the zinc requirement for those consuming a vegetarian diet is approximately 2-fold greater than for those consuming a non-vegetarian diet.

George C. Mihalache

Acronyms

AI Adequate Intake
AMDR Acceptable Macronutrient Distribution Range
BW body weight
DRI Dietary Reference Intake
EAR Estimated Average Requirement
EER Estimated Energy Requirement
LOAEL lowest-observed-adverse-effect level
NOAEL no-observed-adverse-effect level
NRC National Research Council
ND Non determinable
RDA Recommended Dietary Allowance
RNI Recommended Nutrient Intake
SEBR systematic evidence-based review
UL tolerable upper intake level
CHO carbohydrates
DNA deoxyribonucleic acid

Bibliography

1. Dietary Reference Intakes for Water, Potassium, Sodium, Chloride, and Sulfate. The National Academies

2. Dietary Reference Intakes for Calcium, Phosphorous, Magnesium, Vitamin D, and Fluoride (1997). The National Academies

3. Dietary Reference Intakes for Thiamin, Riboflavin, Niacin, Vitamin B6, Folate, Vitamin B12, Pantothenic Acid, Biotin, and Choline (1998). The National Academies

4. Dietary Reference Intakes for Thiamin, Riboflavin, Niacin, Vitamin B6, Folate, Vitamin B12, Pantothenic Acid, Biotin, and Choline (1998). The National Academies

5. Dietary Reference Intakes for Vitamin C, Vitamin E, Selenium, and Carotenoids (2000). The National Academies

6. Dietary Reference Intakes for Vitamin A, Vitamin K, Arsenic, Boron, Chromium, Copper, Iodine, Iron, Manganese, Molybdenum, Nickel, Silicon, Vanadium, and Zinc (2001). The National Academies

Readers fidelity bonus: If you appreciate this book and want to receive the mini-guide of food main nutrients (protein, carbohydrate and fats), send an email to gcmihalache@gmail.com with the title MINIBONUS and you will receive it in the next few days.

Disclaimer: Please specify if you do not want to be informed in advance about my new books.

Kind regards,
George

ABOUT THE AUTHOR

George C. Mihalache published his first book in 2015, his 30 years collection of poetry called "Indescriptible", available in Romanian language. He is also working and is close to finish few other books, with subjects like short fantastic stories, biochemistry or/and a research on the imposter syndrome. With more than 10 years of experience working in Healthcare, he decided to write this book in order to make it easy to understand, ready for everyone with a keen interest in using food supplements.

Printed in Great Britain
by Amazon